Help Me I'm A Hypochondriac!

By Philip Martins

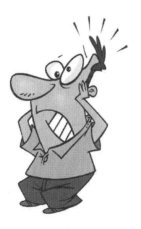

CONTENTS

1 INTRODUCTION

Philip Martins was born in Chichester in the south of England. He is just a normal 36-year-old guy who does normal things like watching all the latest and greatest hit TV shows and playing the odd game, taking a few walks here and there and is really good at freaking out over nothing. He has managed to convince himself many times that he is dying from terrible terminal illnesses over the last eighteen years. Amazingly, he isn't dead yet and is currently exploring the possibility that maybe, just maybe he has a few more years yet. He also worries that by saying such things he'll be struck down by an aneurysm immediately.

He has a forum where people can talk to each other or ask him questions at:

https://www.forum.health-anxiety.com

And he also has a Twitter account that can be used to contact him at:

https://twitter.com/No2Hypochondria (@No2Hypochondria)

2 ABOUT THE BOOK

This is a little something for people to relate to in those dark hours of relentless despair, a few of my own stories and the things I went through when I thought I was dying from illnesses that I imagined and convinced myself I had. Many years ago, when I first realised I was a hypochondriac I would spend pretty much all day of every day on the internet looking for accounts of other peoples self-induced misery in an attempt to cheer myself up.

There was nothing quite like finding out that someone else was going through the same as me and then having a few moments of peace knowing that in fact I wasn't sick. It's also about the times before I realised I was a hypochondriac when I would spend pretty much all day of every day looking for causes to imagined symptoms and learning all the new horrendously painful ways I was going to die that day. Or possibly the day after.

In this little book I will talk about how I got through some of my darker moments but its main purpose is to remind those that suffer from this illness of the mind that they are not alone, that there are people out there who are going through the same thing and more importantly that there are people who have suffered it and no longer do. I am one of those people.

I spent a good three years mostly cooped up in a small room in my mother's house from roughly the age of twenty. During that time, I convinced myself I was due to die from lots of terrible diseases. I remember how I used to see flashes of light when my eyes were closed leading me to believe my retinas were detaching. I remember how if it was a sunny day and the sun went behind a cloud, I started to think I was going blind. There was a time when I read a story about a man in America who had a mastectomy as his brother had breast cancer, I too then had breast cancer. I found bumps on my body that would give me chronic anxiety and they always turned out to be normal body parts.

The issue was I wasn't just checking for problems, I was going out of my way and trying to find them and more often than not I would. I became a panic attack professional which always led to impending heart attacks that, shockingly, never occurred.

There were times when I would venture out of the house usually to my local pub. I'd turn up around midday and sit there sipping beer and whisky until midnight as it was the only way I knew at the time of relieving the anxiety. I was so convinced of my imminent death I would drink myself to oblivion and at that point I couldn't have cared less if I was going to die or not. I'd get angry and decide to punch walls in the bathroom right in front of people and I would burst in to tears in whilst propping up the bar. I'm not sure why I was allowed in there for so long to be honest but it eventually all ended when I pushed one of the regulars too far and he decided to pop my nose. Not exactly my finest hour!

It took me a very long time but eventually I worked out that I wasn't dying or slowly decaying from multiple sclerosis, declining from hereditary motor neurone disease, going blind, suffering from diabetes, on the verge of suffering kidney failure, contracting legionnaires disease, suffering hypoglycaemia, bowel cancer, food poisoning or whatever calamity had befallen me on any given day.

Finding similar stories of people in my situation gave me some comfort. If I was enduring one of my many brain tumour inflictions I would try and comfort myself by searching for brain tumour hypochondria on the internet. I hoped to find an article or something where a guy or gal would tell a story about how they suffered my symptoms related to health anxiety when in reality there was nothing wrong with them at all.

Regardless of the disease I was suffering from at the time I rarely found such encouraging pieces of writing and instead I was often told by my favourite search engine that unfortunately that pain behind my eye was actually optic neuropathy. At the same I would also be politely informed that optic neuropathy is commonly caused by multiple sclerosis or other neurological conditions in people under forty, and as I was only twenty at the time you can imagine how over the moon I was.

Now if you just read that last paragraph and suddenly have a pain in your eye then forget about it. You don't have anything wrong with your eyes, you have something wrong with your brain and we'll go in to that. I should mention that I am not a doctor or some kind of expert, I'm just a guy who went through it all and wants to write down what I experienced and what I learned from it all.

So now that we're friends you and me, let me tell you about my journey of hypochondria. I hope you can read some of my experiences and see in yourself just how ridiculous we both are. Take comfort knowing you are not alone and rest assured that if you really want to you can get though it and see yourself through to the other side.

3 How to Tell if You Are a Hypochondriac

There are a few ways to determine that you may have health anxiety. The best way I learned was to go to my doctor and tell him what was going through my head on a daily basis but it took me three years to get to that point. If this hypochondria business is something new to you and you're not sure if it's all in your mind, or if you really are convinced that you are dying from something nasty and it can't be all in your head then there are some questions you can ask yourself.

Try to answer the following honestly:

- Have you had a headache that has had you convinced that it is a brain tumour?

- Have you had chest pains that have led you to believe you have something wrong with your heart?

- Have you found a rash that you linked to something like meningitis?

- Have you had a cold that wasn't just a cold but a sign of something more sinister?

- Are you very aware of every sensation in your body?

- Do you suffer from many aches and pains or other symptoms that you think could be an illness or medical condition?

- Do you check your body for signs of disease?

- Do you think you have a particular disease that you could detect at home like testicular or breast cancer, but are too afraid to check in case you find something?

- Do you often seek reassurance from those close to you about your health?

- Do you avoid TV shows, films or articles with medical themes?

- If you hear about a disease do you then worry that you have it?

- Do you visit the doctor often?

- When you visit the doctor and they tell you nothing is wrong, do you worry they have missed something?

- Do you find yourself online constantly looking up information on diseases and illnesses?

- Are you regularly stressed or anxious about your health?

- Do you have a disease in mind above all others that you worry about the most?

- Do you find it difficult to sleep at night due to excessive worrying or awareness of sensations in your body?

- Are you still concerned over a potential disease even though your rational side is telling you it's probably nothing?

As I'm not a medical professional I couldn't tell you exactly, but if you found yourself nodding along to six or more of the above questions then it's possible that you are suffering from hypochondria, or as the cool kids are calling it these days, health anxiety. The good news is that if you grab this thing by the horns you can get over it in not too much time if you are prepared to make some changes in your life, accept you have something wrong with you and seek the help you need. The bad news is that if you carry on the way you are, believing you are sick or are going to get sick, surfing the internet for your next disease or constantly checking for that lump then it is probably going to get worse.

I've done worse and I've done even worse than that and it is not a very nice place to be in. So, before you get to that point, and if you think it's possible that you are suffering from hypochondria, give this a quick read and then make the decision to get your life back by doing the things I did and start regaining control of your life.

Most hypochondriacs know that they are hypochondriacs. If you are reading this then you must know or at least suspect that you are a hypochondriac. So why is it that if you are aware that you are a hypochondriac that you constantly feel the physical symptoms of an imagined illness? The key word here is anxiety.

There is an awful lot of science in the explanation of anxiety and how it can affect the body physically. Not being a medical science type myself I can't possibly begin to write in massive detail what is going on in the background between your brain and your body, but I can explain it in basic terms that I forced myself to understand when I realised I was a worrier.

The actual cause of health anxiety varies from person to person and is still not entirely understood though there are a few possible explanations. Some of these include physical or sexual abuse, cyberchondria, a parent that was overly concerned about their health or serious illness or death in friends or family members. It is also possible as was in my case that health anxiety is a symptom of depression, or it could be possible that depression develops as a result of health anxiety and thereby exacerbating the problem.

It took me a long time to realise that actually it was anxiety that was causing a lot of my symptoms. If you are constantly stressed out about your health and causing yourself anxiety then you are placing your body under stress. This stress can then manifest itself physically.

A perfect example is multiple sclerosis, an illness I have "suffered" many times in my life. Let's say you've got your hypochondria hat on and your current condition is MS. One of the symptoms of MS is muscle spasms which unfortunately is also a symptom of anxiety. So there you are sitting down and watching the television and out of the blue you feel a slight twitch in your left leg. Your stress levels go up, the twitching continues and the more it continues the more you think you have MS. Rinse, repeat, panic.

Add to that the fact there are an awful lot of symptoms besides twitching that relate to the muscles alone and you have the perfect recipe. A few examples are pins and needles, weakness, tingling, tension and general aches and pains. For extra fun you can also combine them to create additional misery such as painful twitches in your muscles, one of my all-time favourites and highly recommended! And this is just your muscles we're talking about, there are a bucket load of different symptoms related to all parts of the body that can relate to different illnesses.

Another example is the brain tumour, a classic for the hypochondriac connoisseur. Headaches and dizziness and perhaps migraines, shooting or stabbing pains across the scalp or brain zaps can all be translated in to a brain tumour for the fledgling hypochondriac but again they are all symptoms of an anxiety disorder.

Perhaps have you been suffering from heart palpitations that must mean you have heart disease or are about to have a heart attack? Are you having trouble speaking? Are your words slurring or are you having coordination problems with your mouth and tongue? Is it motor neurone disease? No, it's anxiety. What about crazy thoughts, are you about to go insane? Anxiety.

Are you going to the toilet every ten minutes because of bladder cancer? No, it's because you suffer from anxiety. Is the throat cancer causing that choking sensation? Probably not. Do you feel like you are going to pass out? Is the floor moving from underneath your feet? Must be neurological. Or it could be the other thing.

Racing heart, tight chest, shaking, shooting pains, brain fog, tinnitus and other strange non-existent sounds, finding it hard to breathe, memory problems, a dream like feeling, trapped in a world of slow motion, chronic fatigue, metal taste in your mouth, dry mouth, IBS. Does your tongue twitch? Is your skin itching? Sensitive to light too? What about those little spots you see when you look up?

Think about it. Each one of those symptoms I have listed is a symptom of anxiety. If you looked hard enough the chances are you would find a potentially terminal illness with each one of those symptoms. It's worth pointing out that tiny little list is but a fraction of the potential symptoms you can suffer because of anxiety. And all of them are there to get you even more worked up, get you more anxious and give you more hypochondria fuel.

As I've already said, hypochondria tends to be a symptom. The cause isn't clear but a good place to start is anxiety and depression. Once you can get your head around that fact you can start to look at ways of dealing with the source of your hypochondria, and there are many ways to do that.

As for me, my own journey to the dark side started when I had to spend the night at my dad's place and my sister had claimed the only spare bed in the house. As such I was relegated to the uncomfortable sofa with the dog who somehow by the morning had me perched on the edge whilst he lorded it up like a king with all the space. The day after was the day that I woke up with what to this very moment is still the worst headache of my life. It wasn't just your usual run of the mill take a couple of pills and move on type of headache; it was this all-encompassing band of pain than ran all the way round from temple to temple.

At first, I didn't worry about it too much and all was good. I assumed I had slept in an awkward position or maybe I just hadn't drunk enough water the day before and was dehydrated and so I carried on with my day as usual thinking all would be well and it would go away. The following day when I woke up in my own bed the headache remained but still, I wasn't too bothered by it. I had a driving lesson that day and I had been working hard in my new job as a precision engineer the last few weeks and generally had a lot going on, I was tired and very much looking forward to the weekend and thought a couple of days rest and lots of water would make everything right again.

I can't remember the exact time frame as it was such a long time ago but after about three or four weeks I was still waking up with the headache. My sleeping was beginning to suffer, I was finding it harder to concentrate on various things and I was getting to a point where I generally just couldn't be bothered any more. I was beginning to worry about my headache a lot.

Besides the band of pain that was ever present I was getting strange pains on the top of my head that to this day I still couldn't explain very well. But if I was to try, I would say it was like someone had stuck a screwdriver in to my skull and twisted it until it made my right eye twitch and I was wincing involuntarily. I would move my head to the left and downwards as if in an attempt to try and move away from this pain. It wouldn't last long, a few seconds at most but it was happening frequently. This and the never-ending crushing sensation combined had started to take its toll on me.

I was moving in to a perpetual state of nervousness and was becoming increasingly negative, clearly there was something horribly wrong with me. There was no other explanation for it. I started playing a game where I would wake up and make a bet with myself as to how much pain I would suffer during the coming day. Eventually I went to the doctor where I was told it was a tension headache and I was prescribed some pills to help relax the muscles.

After a couple more weeks, maybe two months in total by this point I was starting to feel very tired and despondent. The tablets the doctor had prescribed hadn't worked and I had run out of them a few days prior and I hadn't gone back to the doctor for another check-up, I couldn't be bothered and so I just carried on getting up and going to work. I'm not sure when it happened, but I remember things started to seem darker.

I would walk outside in to the fresh air and it was almost like it wasn't real, there was a fog in my brain and a grey tinge on the world. If there was a bright object nearby, I couldn't look directly at it. If a white car was close or driving past, I had to look in the other direction as it literally blinded me, and if I had looked at it then it would take a few seconds for my eyes to readjust to the greyness. I used to try and tell people it was like someone had opened up my head, filled it with thick black oil and feathers and closed it back up.

Depression was beginning to set in and the next three years of my life were about to begin.

'My eyes, look at my eyes mum!'

Running as fast as I could down the stairs, I went charging up to my mother who was cooking one of her fine home cooked meals. I went right up to her face and pointed out the obvious difference between the size of my pupils.

'Seriously mum I know it's a brain tumour, I just looked it up on the internet and everything!'

She laughed at me and told me I was just being a hypochondriac. It probably didn't help that a few nights before I had gone and told her I was having some kind of a fit because I couldn't stop shaking. What she didn't realise was that obviously the shaking was just a precursor or symptom of the brain tumour that was now developing. But my mum, bless her, was more interested in peeling potatoes than the fact her only son was about to die. I felt sick and was literally waiting for the projectile vomiting to start as I had read not too long ago that was also a symptom of a brain tumour.

The frustration! I walked away and had a good look in the mirror in the living room making sure my nose wasn't a million miles away from smashing the thing to pieces. But I couldn't see the difference in the lounge so went back upstairs to the bathroom where I'd made my life ending discovery. Sure enough there it was, my right pupil was bigger than my left. I felt dizzy and depersonalised, boiling hot but shivering, scared and exhausted. It was well in to the evening and dinner was almost ready.

I couldn't help but bemoan the fact that I hadn't discovered this in the morning when I could have made an appointment with my doctor and he could have started the process of booking me in for scans. Instead I was now going to have to go to bed and slowly watch the time go by until 8am which was when I could make my appointment. So, I ate my nice home cooked meal and slowly took myself back upstairs to where my computer was so I could continue my research.

By about 11pm I was almost ready to cry. I had been having a sustained panic attack for a good few hours now and the headache was in full swing and adding fuel to the already burning fear that had completely taken over me. I'm not really sure what I did for the rest of the night, knowing me back then I probably went down the local shop and bought some beers to calm me down as at the time it was my way of dealing with it. On a side note, try not to get drunk to calm yourself when you have an anxiety problem as it makes things a lot worse, but I'll touch on that later.

So, the morning came and I made one final check just to be sure I'd seen what I thought I'd seen and yes it was still there. I made my appointment with the doctor and when the time came, off I went to tell my tale of woe.

I'm not one hundred percent sure but it's possible the doctor told me what he told me whilst trying his hardest to suppress a smile.

'If your pupils are different sizes and it's related to a brain tumour, you probably only have about fifteen minutes left to live.'

I can't remember the rest of the conversation but it's irrelevant. I had survived the last fourteen or so hours with my crazy pupil dilation and I was utterly perplexed. Relieved at the same time, but very confused. So off I went back home with my tail between my legs feeling a bit stupid but also with that brief period of calm that always followed after I'd been told by a doctor that it was nothing and I was going to live a while longer.

It was always the same after I'd been to a doctor. I would have a couple of hours of no anxiety, I'd have a good laugh at myself and be in a pretty good mood. I'd switch the computer on and carry on my search looking for other hypochondriac stories knowing that I was well and nothing immediately bad was going to happen to me. The only problem was it would never last for long.

This time it was a little different though, I had a visible sign in my eyes and the doctor had basically told me that my poor mother would already be calling the coroner and having my dead body removed from the house if I had what I thought I had. So, I looked in the mirror again this time really close, really really close. The crazy pupil dilation was still there but the doctor had told me that there was nothing. I looked at my left eye and then my right, then my left again and once more my right. I knew I was being silly, and as my mum later pointed out it wasn't possible for me to look at both pupils at the same time so how could I possibly be sure that one was bigger than the other.

Fair point mum.

So what was it? Well, after a closer inspection with a more rational mindset I noticed that the white frame of the bathroom cabinet on the wall reflected perfectly in to my left eye around the pupil and made it appear smaller than it actually was.

Yep.

That is how irrational I was and how I imagine a lot of hypochondriacs are. There was no reasoning with me back then when I was in that state and now, I can see it clearly and often feel utterly embarrassed by it all. One day you will look back on your crazy moments and want to sink in to hole somewhere but believe me it's much better being embarrassed now than it was being an emotional wreck back then.

My mother still remembers a lot of my dying moments as does my sister. The same goes for my father for that matter and some of my friends too. It makes me cringe to think some of the things I've said to people in the past and sometimes I still think of those moments I had and I hope that they have forgotten most if not all of them. But each person reacted differently to my little episodes, some were supportive and some were dismissive. Sometimes people would understand or at least they would say that they understood but I doubt any of them ever really did. I imagine it is incredibly hard work knowing or living with a hypochondriac or someone who has anxiety or is depressed.

There are many things to consider here if you suffer. There a lot of different feelings and emotions and lots of different thoughts towards people around you. There are times when you feel as if you're a burden dragging people down with you, or a feeling that people just don't really care. Sometimes you may want to talk to people about your problems to help yourself feel better and when you finally find someone that does listen you worry that they are just nodding along with you to keep you happy or telling you what they think you need to hear.

The negative mindset that hypochondriacs can adopt influence greatly their perception of people's reactions and they over analyse things or create scenarios that aren't real. Or at least that's how it was for me.

My mum had very little time for me when I was ill and she would often tell me to just get over it and get on with things. This would make me so angry to the point that sometimes I wished I would develop a genuine illness just so that I could throw it at her and tell her I told you so. But now I think back and I think it's important to bear in mind that unless someone has been where we have been then they can never truly understand what it is like. Nobody can.

I have a friend whose arrogance towards mental health infuriates me beyond belief. I am so much better now but to this day I am still prone to anxiety and on the odd occasion where I have succumbed to panic attacks in front of him, he pulls a face and tells me I need to sort myself out because there is nothing for me to panic over. I did once manage to sit him down and he listened for a good twenty minutes as I explained that there doesn't need to be a source of panic for an attack to happen and that it's a fight or flight response with nothing for it to respond to. He still doesn't understand and I doubt that he ever will.

Interestingly this same friend not too long ago went off to a party and drank a very large quantity of alcohol. A couple of days later he confessed that he was on the verge of ringing me the day after the party because his head was spinning, his heart felt like it was about to burst out of his chest as it was beating so fast and he felt like he was about to die. When I told him that it was probably a panic attack brought on by excessive drinking he just turned around and gave an incredibly stubborn 'don't be stupid, I had nothing to panic about'. The fact I had even mentioned it might have been panic attack made him angry because to him it's not possible to panic over nothing. He refuses to consider the possibility.

Even after I'd explained it all to him, he still couldn't see it. Maybe it wasn't a panic attack, I don't know, but it sure sounded like one. The point of all this is as we all know mental health still has a stigma attached to it and most likely if you are suffering from hypochondria you will encounter people who will just tell you to stop being stupid and to get over it.

But I think now having been there we can't expect people to suddenly stop what they are doing and automatically be supportive and understand what we are going through as much as they shouldn't expect us to suddenly jump up and brush off what is clearly a problem.

Being a hypochondriac can be a lonely journey but it doesn't matter, the only person you need in this fight is you. You will pick up allies such as the doctor as you take the fight to the illness and eventually you will win. Don't be disheartened if those close to you disappoint you with their lack of support, it's not their fault that they don't understand and you should try to not get angry with them if you feel they aren't doing their best to help you.

All that said though I would encourage you to try and find someone to talk to, someone who is willing to listen without judgement even if they can't offer you advice. Now there is one person I would suggest you definitely talk to above all others, someone who you've probably been bothering for a while now but for all the wrong reasons. Go and see the doctor and tell them everything that's going on in your head.

Apart from going to see the doctor what else can we begin to do to kill the hypochondriac in us and start getting our lives back together? I can't pretend that I am going to write some gospel here that by the time you have finished reading is going to have you running down the street screaming I'm cured and I'm free and high fiving random people you meet, but hopefully it will help to give you the confidence to take the first step to getting better. And getting better is what this is all about. I've managed to do it so now it's your turn to do it. So do it!

One of the worst things you can do when you have a symptom that you think is caused by an illness is try to ignore it. Distracting yourself in the midst of a panic attack or an episode of anxiety is a good way to overcome the immediate effects of such a thing, but by distracting yourself from say a pain in your stomach is actually just another way of focusing on it. If you are sitting there telling yourself it's nothing and carrying on with what you are doing, you know yourself that you are ignoring it on purpose and are thinking 'I'm doing this to distract myself from the pain and I know I'm doing it distract myself from the pain, it's not working!'.

The next time you feel a pain or a sensation in your body don't try and distract yourself from it, instead take some time to analyse it. As we've already said it let's work with stomach pain as an example. Let's say you're going about your business as usual and you've been worrying about your stomach for a while now and in the back of your mind you've already decided that it's probably stomach cancer. Suddenly you feel the familiar twinge or the pain you've had a few times over the past week and the worry starts to rise, your brain races, you're pulled in to anxiety and the obsession begins. Instead of going off the rails, sit down if you can and close your eyes, regulate your breathing and try to relax yourself.

Think about the pain in your stomach and start trying to rationalise with yourself. Think of all the other things that can cause stomach pain and go through them one by one. If you prefer then you can write down all the things you know of that can cause discomfort in that area. Remind yourself that as you suffer from health anxiety you are enhancing the awareness of that area of your body and are feeling it more than a non-sufferer would.

Now think about how stomach pain can be caused by a whole range of different things, so instead of jumping to cancer consider the fact that it could just be indigestion, gas or trapped wind. It could be that you pulled a muscle without realising it a few days prior by moving awkwardly or maybe you coughed too hard, two things that can happen without you even noticing. It could be a virus that will pass in a few days or it could be irritable bowel syndrome. It could be nothing and it's simply a symptom of being alive, we all get aches and pains from time to time and it's just one of those things.

When I started analysing my thoughts like this, I would also think about the symptoms that I didn't have. For example, I wasn't vomiting, my skin wasn't turning yellow and I wasn't having trouble swallowing food. I didn't feel sick, I wasn't frequently burping and I didn't have pains in my chest. I coupled this knowledge with the fact that stomach cancer is one of the rarer forms of cancer. In the United Kingdom where I live there is a population of over sixty million people and of those sixty million people roughly seven thousand are diagnosed with stomach cancer each year, or 0.0116% of the total population.

When you start thinking in these terms you are trying to deal with the feelings that are accompanied with the pain. The objective is to remove the feelings of fear and by doing that the negative thoughts begin to take care of themselves. In the end I began to realise that the chances of me having cancer were extremely remote and made me feel sorry for the poor souls that had it. Here I was freaking out and making something of nothing when there were people actually going through it for real.

There are other examples we can use too. Brain tumours and multiple sclerosis were the two things I often came back to and these can easily be explained away using calm and logic. As far as headaches go, did you know that there are over two hundred different types of headache and that these are split in to primary headaches and secondary headaches. 90% of all headaches are primary, are benign and not caused by disease. These headaches can be caused by dehydration, alcohol, poor posture, skipped meals, sinus problems, stress and anxiety among other things.

The other 10% of headaches, secondary headaches, are caused by problems that affect the nerves in your head. The causes of these types of headache can range from dehydration, dental problems, overuse of pain medication, cold or flu, sinusitis, MSG found in some foods, wearing a bike helmet or a pair of sunglasses too long and, wait for it... panic and anxiety!

Multiple sclerosis can be something as simple as having been sat in the same position for too long. I had a lot of bouts of "MS" when I was ill, and sitting still for too long was what caused most of it. After not moving for a long time I would go to scratch an itch or something on my leg and realise that it was partially numb. I'd then scratch my other leg in the same spot and test to see if it was more sensitive which it always was. Then I'd scratch my left leg again, then my right and so it went on and on and on.

I've probably spent three days in total of my life scratching my arms and legs to see if one side was numb or more sensitive than the other, always thinking it was MS. Tingling sensations can also be caused by vitamin deficiencies, alcohol, injury, pinched nerves and anxiety. And as we already know anxiety can cause fatigue, vision problems, bladder control problems, muscle spasms, balance and co-ordination problems, issues with thinking clearly, all symptoms of MS.

I have my own example of how I dealt with something that one day may affect me although it's very unlikely. My grandmother passed away from motor neurone disease towards the end of my illness and as you would expect this caused me a lot of stress. Not only because she was someone who I had known and loved my whole life, but also because being an idiot I looked up the disease online and discovered that MND has a hereditary link and that fact then sent me in to overdrive.

Overnight I suddenly had every symptom you can link to the disease. I had already read about it previously before she was diagnosed so I was well prepared to go full hypochondriac on this one. As soon as my mum told me that the doctor had found a quiver on her tongue and to expect the worst, my own tongue started twitching almost immediately. But it was her that was going through it and eventually she passed.

As it stands today about 10% of people diagnosed with MND have a familial link. There are about 5,000 people living in the UK that have MND and it affects two in every 100,000 people. It doesn't scare me at all.

So now in future when you get hit by panic caused by a symptom, be cool and calm and tell yourself that you are fine. Learn to understand that the thing you think you have is one of many different possibilities and remember that you have health anxiety. Because once you can control the emotions, the actual thought of something bad happening to you passing through your mind isn't really that bad and after you have learned that control you can observe the thought and then let it go on its way.

7 ANXIETY AND PANIC ATTACKS

Easily one the worst and most challenging parts of being a hypochondriac are the panic attacks. To be honest without them I don't think being a hypochondriac would be such a big deal. These nasty horrible things are inexplicable to someone who has never had to suffer one and I wouldn't wish them on my worst enemy. When I speak to people about my battle with hypochondria, I often talk to them about the madness of it all with some humour and a smile, but these things... wow.

My smile fades, my head shakes and I often give a scratch of the beard as I contemplate the sheer horror of it all. They really are the stuff of nightmares, although in my opinion panic attacks make nightmares seem like sweet tales of fluffy bunnies having a picnic in a meadow surrounded by rainbows while singing songs about sweets and chocolate covered cupcakes.

The good news is that these bad boys can be controlled and can be as brief as three minutes. The bad news is if you are new to panic attacks and don't know how to control them, they can last several hours up to several days or more. It's not uncommon for people who experience their first panic attack to end up in accident and emergency at the hospital.

My first panic attack happened as I was watching television at my mum's house with a friend. I didn't know what a panic attack was at the time and having never experienced one I almost completely lost the plot when it started. It began, as most of my future attacks did, with what's called a brain zap.

For those who don't know what a brain zap is, it feels as if you have had a bolt of energy rush through your brain and it's like the world goes out of focus and then comes back in a split second. It can also be described as an electric shock type sensation or a jolt and isn't too different from the odd feeling you sometimes get as you're falling asleep and suddenly feel as if you are falling. It's also a symptom of anxiety and so is part of the whole hypochondria/anxiety/panic attack cycle.

As soon as that happened to me my heart rate upped itself dramatically, my stomach turned, my head started spinning and I started shaking. I had been obsessing over my health for a while at this point and this new horrible feeling was the thing I had been expecting for a while, my final throes in this mortal coil as my dying body was finally giving in to whatever disease I had at that time.

Barely holding myself together I stood up and held my head in my hands as this wave of terror came over me. I ended up asking my friend to leave the house which he did and then I took myself up the stairs and laid down on my bed. I was staring at the ceiling one second and rolling around on the bed the next, then I was on all fours gasping for air and then followed up by curling in to a foetal position and bursting in to tears. It lasted for about two hours.

I have never felt fear like it. The thoughts that can run through your head during a panic attack are irrational and scary and often add to the fear. I was thinking of my family and how I would never see them again, how I was only young and I hadn't done anything of any note and the fact my bedroom was a mess and how embarrassing it was going to be for someone to have to come and clear it out after I was dead. If you have found yourself feeling like this at some point in your life and you still aren't sure what was going on and you are still alive to tell the tale then chances are you have suffered a panic attack.

One of the hardest things about panic attacks is trying to be calm. If you are mid panic your heart is racing but because your heart is racing your panic continues to rise. It is a viscous cycle and as I said it is truly one of the most horrific things that can happen to a human being. So what is going on and what can we do about it?

As animals we are primed to survive and a part of survival is being able to identify and react to immediate danger almost instantly. Our bodies respond to danger by initiating something called the fight or flight response.

This reaction to perceived danger by the body is a very useful thing to have and is essential to human survival. There is a complicated physiological response produced by the human body when a threat is present and I'm not going to go in to great detail about the chain of events that lead to a fight or flight response, but the upshot of it all is that there is a large release of adrenaline in to the blood stream that prepares the body for action, be it to fight a threat or to run away from it.

So, what happens when this response is triggered by something like a chest pain or a brain zap? What good is this response to us when there is nothing for us to run from or to fight? Absolutely no good whatsoever. That brain zap that I had scared me and presented what my brain perceived to be as danger. My body reacted by initiating the fight or flight response but of course I had nothing to act upon. My heart rate increased, I began breathing quicker and I started perspiring. Because there was no need for me to react physically, I was left sitting in a chair with a bunch of hormones and adrenaline raging through my system telling my muscles to get a move on and get out of the way of whatever was coming, or alternatively to give a good kicking. Either way there wasn't much for me to do and the result was panic.

Once the process is started it is difficult to bring under control, especially in hypochondriacs where the physical effects of a panic attack can be translated in to a potentially life-threatening situation whereby you think that the heart attack you've been expecting is about to come and get you. Your heart rate increases further and fuels that fear even more and so your body keeps you on the edge until the "danger" is passed.

It's important to remember that if this happens to you then nothing bad will come of it in the end. As far as I know no one has ever died from a panic attack and I'm pretty sure you aren't going to be the first one to go down in history. It's worth remembering that this physiological response is the bodies way of protecting itself and so it isn't about to go and do something that is going to kill you.

There are a fair few symptoms to look out for during a panic attack. If you feel the beginnings of one creeping up on you try and take a second to observe what is happening in your body. I know this isn't an easy thing to do with an irrational mind and you might be wondering how but if you start practising now you can take control of these attacks.

Even now I don't always get a grip on my own before they take hold as quite often the thought of having a panic attack will make me have a panic attack. But if you experience symptoms such as palpitations, sweating, a feeling of choking, numbness or tingling, dizziness, the feeling that you really are about to die or that you feel like you are losing control or going insane then you know it's a panic attack. It's not death and you can control it.

We can start to learn how to control these attacks by learning more about them. With knowledge you can begin to identify an attack and like I do now you can shut the attack down before it even begins and you should consider this to be your first line of defence.

However do not be disheartened if you don't manage to control yourself even though you know what's about to happen isn't going to be fatal, I still don't manage it sometimes but if we cross the barrier and the adrenaline gets the better of us then we need to accept that it's happening and move on to a different strategy which is to regulate your breathing and do your best to carry on doing what you are doing as if nothing is wrong.

Our instinct is to breathe faster when we are first hit with panic. We breathe deep and then start to take short sharp breaths increasing the amount of carbon dioxide in the blood and this is something that is thought to contribute to a panic attack. If you begin to feel your breath becoming erratic then try to control it by breathing in through the nose, holding for a few seconds and then breathe out through the mouth pursing your lips. After this pause for a couple of seconds then repeat the process. Do your best to stop yourself from breathing too deeply too quickly and maintain control.

Another thing you can try is tensing different muscles in your body and then relaxing them. Begin with your feet by tensing the muscles for a few seconds then release the tension when you are breathing out. Do this and then move up the body combining it with the breathing exercise above, not only is this helping your body to relax but you are also taking the focus away from panic and it is preventing you from going in to a deeper attack.

Physical sensations aren't the only thing that can trigger an attack as your own thoughts can also be responsible. This is my main source of attacks these days as I tend not to suffer from phantom symptoms any more, instead I will suddenly remember that I have something to do the following day that is already making me nervous for example, and this will give me the brain zap which then makes me prone to attack. If you suffer from this problem then try to observe the thought and let it pass. You may feel that sensation in your stomach which can rise up and lead to an attack but just let it go over you by closing your eyes and taking a deep controlled breath.

I know you may be thinking that sounds impossible, I used to read about people who just observed their thoughts and wondered what on earth they were talking about and doubted it was even possible. But it is and now that I am able to do it myself, I can understand what they were trying to say, and you will too.

As well as the above I would suggest leaving yourself things to do if you think you will be unable to control an attack in the future. Try leaving a pack of cards nearby and if you feel one coming on play a game such as solitaire. Or leave a crossword book somewhere for you to solve. If you have a games console then switch it on and play something you enjoy. The aim is to distract yourself from what's happening and letting yourself calm down.

Eventually when all is said and done you will get to a point where you will be able to bring yourself under control quickly. After an attack you may feel extremely tired as your body has just endured a great deal of stress. If it's appropriate then go and have a lie down and have a sleep.

Asides from cure one of the best methods is prevention as is the case in most things in life. There are a few things you can do now to help stop anxiety and hopefully by doing so you can decrease the chances of having an attack. The first of these is to look at your diet. It took me a very long time to realise that what I was putting in to my body was affecting my moods.

One of the first changes I made was to cut out the coffee, or anything that contained a high level of caffeine. It was painful to do as I loved my morning coffee and if I'm honest I quite liked energy drinks as well. Caffeine triggers the release of adrenaline which is the source of the fight or flight response, so in a way you're drinking a cup of freshly brewed panic attack and that's a bad cup to be drinking.

Caffeine has also been shown to inhibit the levels of serotonin, a compound that is thought to affect your mood and behaviour, your appetite and your sleep among other things. A lack of serotonin is believed by some to lead to the things that are discussed in this book such as depression, anxiety, panic attacks and as a result as is in our case could lead to or contribute towards hypochondria. Caffeine can also keep you awake and you need good sleep to help keep you in a positive mood, so as hard as it may be, I would suggest this be the first thing you change if you are a regular consumer. For me this was by far the best thing I did to help calm me down.

Another painful life choice you can make is to cut out the alcohol. This for me was one of the hardest things I did as I often used alcohol to calm myself down, especially when I was very anxious or having a panic attack. Yes, the immediate effect is calmness and I was often elated, but as soon as I felt the effects wearing off, I would grab another six pack, another bottle of wine or worse I'd go for whiskey or vodka. I spent probably a year of my life drinking every day just to stave off the anxiety.

I would go through the mornings feeling very nervous and panicky and as soon as midday came, I would hit the booze and carry on drinking until I passed out, usually in the early evenings. I would be sure to leave something to drink lying around for when I inevitably woke up at 1am just so I was able to get back to sleep. It was a pretty awful thing to go through and I have no idea how I managed it for a year without killing myself though I had my fair share of accidents and made myself look very stupid on many occasions.

Drinking excessive amounts of alcohol can trigger anxiety, especially the next day as it begins to leave the body. I found the phrase "hangxiety" online once and it is definitely the best description you can use! Alcohol is also a depressant so again it brings about all the problems we need to deal with in order to become panic free and ultimately get rid of hypochondria. So, if you like to drink then you should look at cutting alcohol out of your life or at least reduce it. A beer or a glass of wine here and there probably isn't going to make much difference but if you find you feel edgy after a drink then maybe it's time to put the bottle down.

If you can combine the above suggestions and at the same time start drinking lots of water then you can make a really big difference. It's well known that most of us don't drink enough water, and when we become dehydrated our bodies can interpret this as a threat to our survival and so can cause us to feel anxious and panicky.

Water is one of the most important things we can put in to our bodies as it transports all kinds of hormones and nutrients to the vital organs. I always carry a bottle with me wherever I go, even around the house as it acts as a constant reminder that I need to keep drinking water. It is possible to be dehydrated without realising and often we can interpret being thirsty as a sign of hunger which may lead to snacking between meal times on things such as sweets or sandwiches that we don't really need.

Sweets themselves can cause you to feel tired after the initial sugar rush has worn off and leave you feeling jaded or in a low mood which can increase anxiety. So, if you're a jelly bean addict think about cutting back on the sugars. This goes for cakes too, so put down that Bakewell tart!

Instead of all the stuff that is marketed to us day in day out by companies desperate to make a penny off of us, stick to what humans have been eating since long before the days of advertising. Go to the fresh produce section of the supermarket and start buying fruits and vegetables such as leafy greens, avocados, tomatoes and onions. Stock up on apples, invest in some seeds and buy fresh unadulterated meat. Try to keep anything containing chemicals or anything that's been modified in any way out of your system; it's how the human race has made it this far so why now do we need to ingest all the rubbish we see on the television? And did I mention drink lots of water? Definitely drink lots of water!

If you're a smoker like I was then think about kicking the habit. I know it's a big ask and if you really cannot do it then at least do the diet thing. But smoking is a terrible thing for anxiety and doesn't actually relax us in the way that we think it does. Nicotine increases the heart rate and pushes up the blood pressure which are two physical symptoms that mirror anxiety.

I lost count of how many panic attacks I had when I had my first cigarette of the day and then how I made them worse smoking another one trying to calm down. Of course, the down side of quitting smoking is nicotine withdrawal which itself can cause anxiety. What worked for me was nicotine replacement therapy and over time I slowly decreased my bodies need for nicotine and eventually I quit completely.

Lastly and importantly you should get yourself exercising. I'm not talking about spending a small fortune on signing up to a crazy expensive monthly gym subscription but instead going out for a thirty minute walk each day. This can help to relieve some tension and stress and decrease fatigue. It also helps to increase your appetite so you can appreciate all the new food you can eat and can also help you sleep better which in turn will help you to feel better the next day.

I know a lot of what is written here requires motivation and that isn't an easy thing to come by if you are feeling worried or depressed but you can break all this down in to little step by step changes and gradually you can start to feel better and stop overly worrying. Believe me, if I am capable of making some changes then you certainly are. I was the worst for smoking, drinking and eating cheeseburgers several times a day for many years and once you get started it all becomes quite easy very quickly.

8 CYBERCHONDRIA

We all know the internet is an amazing and wonderful thing that has brought us a new wealth of information to our fingertips, if you can think of it then you can almost certainly find it. The internet has also made becoming a hypochondriac an easy two-step process which can be achieved by anyone with a little computer literacy and a slight disposition towards health worries. The first step is to have a symptom and the second is to search for it.

There are examples of people in the world having a look online for causes of their symptoms and then going on to find out that in fact they were ill and then being cured. That said, if you know you are likely to overreact to any information you may stumble across online as I'm guessing most hypochondriacs are then I cannot stress enough how much you shouldn't go online and look for incorrect answers you most likely don't want to find. Believe me, I speak from experience and you will make your life miserable.

If an individual is suffering from hypochondria it is a fair assumption that on some level the mental health of that person is somewhat compromised. This individual will most likely take the incorrect and irrational view that what they have just read about their symptoms being caused by an illness as true.

You might read that a certain condition presents symptoms of pain in both eyes and that little pain behind just one of your eyes is now behind both, or the numbness in your right hand is now in your left but twice as bad as in the right. That heart attack that's been creeping up on you all morning with those chest pains is now accompanied by that shooting pain in your left arm. These are just examples.

But wait, how do you know it's a shooting pain if it's a heart attack and not a dull constant pain located in a singular spot? Well as you don't know for sure you go ahead and look it up on the internet. Digging a little deeper you soon learn that as well as a pain in your arm, a heart attack can also be accompanied by a pain in your jaw.

Thinking back on it, didn't you have some pain in your jaw when you woke up this morning, or was it last night when you were watching repeats of Friends on Comedy Central? Or was it actually never, but as rationality isn't a strong point of yours at this stage you disregard the fact that you are pretty sure you're a hypochondriac and you just go right ahead and let your brain trigger that fight or flight response and really get the adrenalin pumping.

With your pulse racing and still reeling from the now almost certain heart attack that's bound to be triggered by your 160 beats per minute heart rate, you frantically search for causes of jaw pain relating to heart attacks looking for information. Suddenly at this point you remember from a previous search that jaw cancer is a thing, what if actually it's that? What if it's not a heart attack at all and it's all related to something different?

So off you go looking for symptoms of jaw cancer and before you know it your heart attack is a distant memory. Shaking, sweating and close to tears you put your head in your hands as it spins round and you come to terms with the fact that you now have cancer.

So, it is with every fibre of my being that I ask, no I beg you, never ever look up your symptoms on the internet.

Ever.

For any reason.

No matter how tempted you are to search for answers on the internet I cannot in any stronger terms without using bad language say to you that really shouldn't do it. Even if it's to find something that's non-lethal that matches your symptoms in an attempt to be rational you simply should not do it. It will break you, seriously. Do not do it. It's bad and you're bad if you do it. Don't be bad.

Even now at this very second as I'm writing I've just gone and inadvertently broken my own rule by doing some research causing me to have my own little mini episode.

For a week or so I have been suffering from what may be a cold and I have also had a slight stomach pain from a bug that I picked up no too long ago. Scouring the internet for some facts and figures and not even looking for causes of what's ailing me I came across the headline "Why cancer symptoms can sometimes seem like the flu". And just like that the panic rose up and started to take me.

Luckily, I'm a bit of a legend when it comes to controlling anxiety and I put it down pretty quick as I have had many years of practice. But it's an example of how delicate my own mind is even after years of not suffering.

9 GOING TO THE DOCTOR

Hands down the best thing you can do to cure yourself is going to see a doctor. I finally made the decision to go after several rounds of really bad anxiety. I had convinced myself that I had bladder cancer when in fact all I was doing was drinking about eight cups of coffee every day and running to the toilet every ten minutes. I was also struggling with new challenges. I had become afraid of people knocking on the door and was constantly checking out the window for cars pulling up and seeing who was there.

The last straw came when a salesman knocked on the door and I ran upstairs in tears and hid in a corner on my hands and knees with my head on the floor. I was clutching at my head and grinding my teeth, almost trying to drag the insanity out of my head. I was convinced I was going insane and decided to go see the doctor and tell him everything that was happening to me despite the embarrassment. No more visiting to have an illness confirmed, a straight up confession of a hypochondriac gone too far.

I made the call the next day and made my appointment and went in to see him, sat down in the chair in front of him and started to tell him the whole story. I told him how it had started with a headache that escalated in to a brain tumour. I talked about how my back pain was kidney failure and how my aching muscles were a wasting disease. I mentioned the vision problems that led me to believe that my retina was detaching from my eyes and how the spots I would see had me thinking I had MS. I spoke about how I was drinking to mask the pain. I regaled how I would cook chicken until it was charcoal because I didn't want food poisoning. I told him I rarely went out as I was always too nervous and how I'd lost a lot of my friends and become a recluse.

By the time I had finished speaking I was a nervous wreck and shaking like a leaf. He asked me if I felt nervous right then and I told him I honestly thought I was going mad. After all this time of believing I was on deaths door, finally telling the truth to someone who was actually listening just felt right and, in that moment, I could feel some of the weight lifting off of me. Somehow, I knew I had taken the first step towards a better life and it felt good.

He waved his hand and told me that I wasn't going mad and that I had all the hallmarks of someone that was suffering from depression. I knew he was right. Through all the searching I had done on the internet the word depression had popped up numerous times and yet I had never really taken it seriously, instead always choosing to believe that I was sick. He told me that everything I was experiencing was down to anxiety and that with the right treatment everything was going to be fine. He took the time to book me in for some blood tests anyway just to be sure there really wasn't anything physically wrong with me and a few weeks later all the results came back negative.

In the end he put me on a course of antidepressants and asked me if I'd like to speak to someone, a cognitive behavioural therapist. My first response was to say no, I wasn't too keen on the idea of someone listening to me who is paid to listen as I didn't really think they'd care. As soon as I said it, I suddenly realised who I was talking to, so I made my apology and accepted the offer of cognitive behavioural therapy, or CBT for short. And that was the first day of my recovery, the beginning of the end of my hypochondria.

I left his office and went next door to the pharmacy to pick up my prescription and started my recovery right there and then. I went to the shop on the opposite side of the road and bought a nice sugary energy drink to take my first pill with and almost immediately had a panic attack from the caffeine content. It was awesome.

In the end though and as I said before, that little trip was the best thing I did and above all else is what I would suggest you do first and foremost of all the things I have written here. I had got myself so worked up over all these things and the thought of going to the doctor to tell the truth had always made me feel embarrassed and stupid and I had always thought for some reason that the doctors wouldn't care. So, if you are moping around worrying about a visit to the doctor then please stop. Make that appointment and start your recovery.

I would definitely recommend CBT as a course of action. I was very sceptical to begin with but after a couple of sessions I started to see things differently. My therapist also encouraged me to keep a diary of my thoughts and feelings and my worries. For me personally this didn't work as I needed to update my diary every hour and constantly checking the time and reminding myself to fill in my anxiety diary gave me anxiety. But if your therapist suggests it and it works then stick with it.

Don't be afraid to start the process. Don't worry that if you go that your doctor is going to fob you off. If you go and tell them the truth from start to finish and tell them you think you have health anxiety then they will help you. Once you've taken the first step you can start to implement some of the things we have discussed in this book and bring an end to this unnecessary misery.

There has been some debate over the years at the effectiveness of antidepressants. Some say that they are a complete waste of time or increase the effects of depression, or in some cases can cause suicidal thoughts and actions. Other people swear that they worked for them and wouldn't be where they are today if it wasn't for the pills. Me personally, I fall in to the latter category.

I don't think the antidepressants were completely responsible for my recovery. They worked for me in the sense that they managed to pull me back from the bottomless pit far enough so that I was able to start working on my mind and the way it functioned. With them, I was able to accept that CBT could help and I was able to apply some of the techniques that I had learned. They allowed me to feel positive about the changes I was making to my lifestyle and gave me the belief that how I was beginning to live my life was having a positive effect.

Without that boost and remembering how I used to think things like what's the point, why bother and nothing can help me, I'm not sure if anything I tried would have worked or if I would have even bothered to try and improve myself. When I was at the bottom, I physically couldn't bring myself to do anything about anything let alone step up and try and sort my life out.

Everybody who is suffering from depression is suffering from varying degrees of it. There are mildly depressed people who can muster enough motivation to keep going, and then there are extremely depressed people like I was who, ironically, despite being terrified of dying from an illness felt like if I got hit by a bus and had everything end right there it would have been be the best thing that could have happened.

The most common type of antidepressants are known as selective serotonin reuptake inhibitors or SSRIs. Some of these SSRIs work by increasing the levels of serotonin, a compound produced in the body and believed to contribute to a feeling of well-being and happiness. Other SSRIs work by decreasing the levels of serotonin and others have no effect at all. Yet despite this, varying medications have been shown in some studies to have a similar positive effect leading to the belief that by simply taking action against depression the patient begins to heal themselves.

This has led to some people believing that the tablets themselves aren't responsible for anything and instead the individual creates the belief that they are getting better and begin to do so, or in other words they create the placebo effect. While medication increases the levels of serotonin in the brain, it is disputed by many that depression and it's resulting symptoms are actually caused by a serotonin shortage.

This is a debate that has raged on for years and so I can't tell you what is right and what is wrong. All I can tell you is that for me it worked. Even if it was a placebo and I tricked myself in to thinking that I was feeling better, the end result was that I did feel better. But whether or not you decide to take antidepressants if you are offered them is down to you as an individual. Because of this you need to bear in mind that the pros and cons of medication are down to each person's own experience or beliefs.

So, with all that in mind, what are the most common types of antidepressant and what can they do to make you feel better? And on the flip side, what can they do to make things worse?

All SSRIs do mainly the same thing but have slight differences such as how stimulating they are and how long the drug stays in your system. I was prescribed fluoxetine and it was the only antidepressant that I took as it worked for me right off the bat. Other common antidepressants include citalopram, escitalopram, fluvoxamine, paroxetine and sertraline.

On the positive side of the scale antidepressants can help to improve your sleeping, and a good sleep is key to feeling well and rested the next day. On the flip side SSRIs can increase dreams and their intensity as I can attest to, I had some of the craziest dreams ever when I began my treatment. Of course, where there are dreams there can be nightmares and some users have reported suffering from these regularly after they started medicating themselves.

Other benefits can be pain relief as anxiety begins to subside, improved health in the sense that you are no longer putting your body under constant stress and increasing the risk of developing a real illness somewhere down the line, your work performance can improve and you can socialise better. Your memory can improve and you can think more clearly and new found motivation can help you lead a healthier lifestyle by exercising more.

As well as less serious side effects such as increased appetite, stomach cramps, weight loss, sexual dysfunction, changes in vision and changes in taste and smell, SSRIs have been reported to do more harm than good in some circumstances. One example is that antidepressants can cause a serotonin shortage which can lead to an irregular heartbeat, seizures and unconsciousness. Other people have reported feeling suicidal or have taken to self-harming. Other bad news is that antidepressants may lose their effectiveness after a certain amount of time and there is also a danger of side effects when they are discontinued such as withdrawal.

It's a tricky subject and you should carefully evaluate your situation before starting any course of medication. There are of course other alternatives, natural remedies such as curcumin which some believe to be as effective as fluoxetine. Many types of natural therapy can be bought from shops or online and often don't come with side effects.

When all is said and done, it is up to you if you feel you need a boost to give you the help needed to start being proactive about your anxiety. But for whatever reason the pills gave me the boost I needed and helped me on to where I am today.

11 In the End

It's a sad fact of life that one day no matter how much we worry about it; all of this is going to come to an end. We are all going to die. I decided back then that I didn't really like the idea of laying on my death bed knowing that the end of my life was near and thinking back at how I had wasted it all worrying about the inevitable moment that claims us all.

Do you really want to be eighty years old and in your final moments regretting that you'd wasted all those days in what could have been a happy life? Imagine how angry you will be knowing you could have done a whole lot more but instead chose to panic your days away.

The negative mindset we're trying to beat may well have us think that we're not going to make it to eighty. You might be thinking you know you're going to get sick, and the minute you stop worrying about it is the minute you get that terminal disease. Well maybe one day you will. Maybe I will. Who knows, but what's the point of worrying about it?

Life is too short to be wasted worrying, and the sad fact is the more we worry the more likely we are going to make ourselves ill and the shorter our lives will be. If you are in a constant state of anxiety and frequently panicking then you are breaking your heart, literally. The constant worry is genuinely making your health worse and this is one of the best reasons to bring it to an end.

Today, I don't suffer from hypochondria at all. Not one bit of me worries about my health irrationally. I don't feel any more random sensations or have pins and needles. I no longer have headaches and I don't feel like I'm choking all the time on nothing. I can actually get out of bed before the sun goes down in the afternoon and I have stopped cooking poultry to within an inch of its life. Since my illness I have done some great things like travelling and meeting new people, I've worked in various places and experienced lots of new things.

The funny thing is that despite how horrible the whole thing was I wouldn't change it. I don't wish that it never happened. When you come out the other side things are different and you are certainly a wiser person for the experience. You will see things differently and you will probably find you can empathise with other people much better when they feel down. In a way I think it has made me a better person.

So, remember, no matter how bad it seems now, no matter how convinced you are that you're on your last legs, just remember that you can get over this and you can start doing it right now. Remember that there are people that have been where you are now and then remind yourself that those people aren't there anymore.

I am one of those people, and you will be too!

12 A NOT COMPREHENSIVE LIST OF ANXIETY SYMPTOMS

Anger

Bad taste in mouth

Blanching - Looking pale

Blocked ear feeling

Blurry vision

Blushing

Body Aches/Jolts/Zaps/Shakes/Tremors

Body temperature fluctuations

Brain fog

Brain zaps

Burping

Changes in the voice

Chest - Pain/Tightness

Choking sensation in throat

Co-ordination problems/Clumsiness

Cold chills

Cold or flu like symptoms

Constipation

Cough

Crazy thoughts

Crying

Decreased sex drive

Deja vu

Depth perception feels incorrect

Diarrhoea

Difficulty speaking or moving the mouth

Difficulty swallowing

Dry mouth

Dry or itchy eyes

Easily startled

Emotionally numb

Excess energy

Faintness

Falling sensations

Fatigue

Feeling inexplicably sick

Feeling out of sorts, different, strange

Feeling unreal

Feeling worse in the mornings

Fears of -

  Being in public

  Being overwhelmed

  Dying

  How you are perceived by others

  Impending doom

  Losing control or losing your mind

  Of situations and circumstance

Flashing lights in eyes when closed

Floor is moving under you sensation

Frequent urination

Grinding teeth

Hair loss

Headaches and migraines

Hearing noises when you wake up

Heart palpitations

Hot and cold flushes

Hot and cold hands and feet

Hypersensitivity

IBS

Inexplicable sounds like ringing, humming or fizzing

Intermittent "deafness" in one ear or reduced hearing

Lack of concentration

Lethargy

Memory loss

Metallic tastes and smells

Mixing words when speaking

Mood swings

Motion sickness

Muscles - Twitching/Weakness/Vibrations

Muscle tension

Nausea

Nervous cough

Never ending thinking of the same thing

Nightmares

Numb or tingling hands

Out of breath

Pain

Painful jaw

Panic attacks

Persistent infections

Pins & needles

Racing or pounding heart

Racing thoughts

Ringing ears

Sadness

Seeing flashes of light or stars

Sensation of forced breathing

Sensitive to light

Shaking

Shooting or stabbing pains –
Face/Head/Neck/Chest/Arms & Legs

Skin - Itchy/Prickly/Crawly/Burning/Numbness/Pins
& Needles

Skipped heart beats

Slow motion feelings

Spasms in the oesophagus

Spots in vision

Stiff neck

Sugar cravings

Sweating at night

Tight scalp

Tongue -
Tingly/Burning/Aching/Sore/Numb/Twitching/Itchy

Unable to digest new information
Unreachable itch in ear
Vibration in fingers, toes, hands, arms and legs
Vomiting
Waking up in a panic attack
Yawning...

And just about anything else you can think of.

Made in the USA
San Bernardino, CA
23 November 2019